How to Apply Make Up Like In the Movies

Over 100 Tips and Hints On How to Apply Make Up

By: Jasinth H. Gooden

9781631871757

PUBLISHERS NOTES

Disclaimer – Speedy Publishing, LLC

This publication is intended to provide helpful and informative material. It is not intended to diagnose, treat, cure, or prevent any health problem or condition, nor is intended to replace the advice of a physician. No action should be taken solely on the contents of this book. Always consult your physician or qualified health-care professional on any matters regarding your health and before adopting any suggestions in this book or drawing inferences from it.

The author and publisher specifically disclaim all responsibility for any liability, loss or risk, personal or otherwise, which is incurred as a consequence, directly or indirectly, from the use or application of any contents of this book.

Any and all product names referenced within this book are the trademarks of their respective owners. None of these owners have sponsored, authorized, endorsed, or approved this book.

Always read all information provided by the manufacturers' product labels before using their products. The author and publisher are not responsible for claims made by manufacturers.

This book was originally printed before 2014. This is an adapted reprint by Speedy Publishing, LLC with newly updated content designed to help readers with much more accurate and timely information and data.

Speedy Publishing, LLC

40 E Main Street,

Newark

Delaware

19711

Contact Us: 1-888-248-4521

Website: http://www.speedypublishing.com

REPRINTED Paperback Edition: ISBN: 9781631871757

Manufactured in the United States of America

DEDICATION

This book is dedicated to my loving family. They support me no matter what I do and they encourage me when I am not totally confident about what I am doing.

TABLE OF CONTENTS

Chapter 1- How to Care for Your Skin

At some point in your life, you will start to reflect on your aging. It might be a line that shows up or a gray hair that catches your eye as you look in the mirror. Either way, though, you will see it and it will be time to start considering the implication of growing old. You don't want to just lie down and take it, though, do you? The number one way you can fight the effects of aging is by taking care of your skin. By taking the proper measures to care for your skin from head to toe, you will be able to reverse some of those effects of aging while at the same time improving the health of your skin as well.

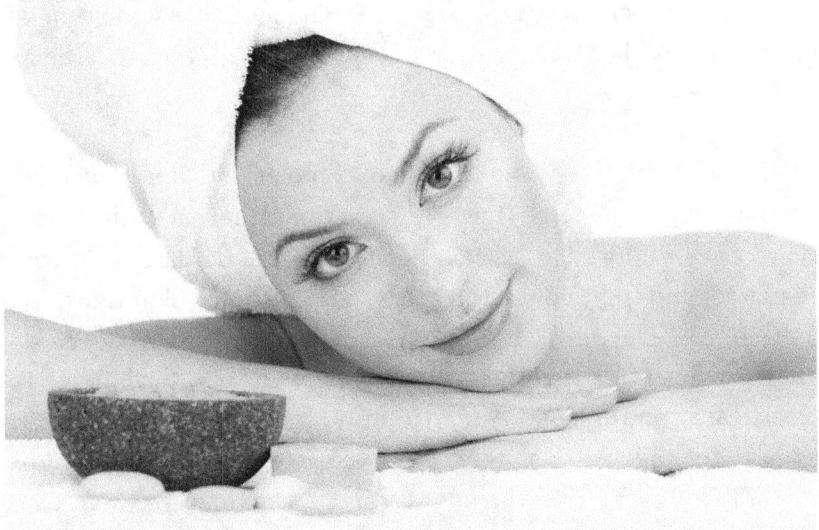

What steps should you take then? The best way to remember is that you have to keep with your "ABC's" when caring for your skin from head to toe. "A" is for anti-aging cream, "B" is for blemish control, and "C" is for collagen. If you keep those three words in mind, you will be well on your way to proper skin care and reversal of those wrinkles associated with aging. Each word is a reminder about an important step in the skin care and age reversing process.

"A" is for anti-aging cream, and that is an incredibly important step in the care of your skin. Hopefully you were properly hydrating and caring for your skin before that first wrinkle. If you weren't, though, once you see that little aging sign it is time to spring into action. Waiting or ignoring the wrinkle is the worst thing you can do. Once you see a sign at all, application of a quality anti-aging cream will possibly stop new lines from forming while getting rid   of the one or two wrinkles that have shown up already.

Though anti-aging creams are not miracle drugs or fountains of youth, they do actually help. They are made up of vital vitamins and nutrients that science has proven to rejuvenate skin. Look for an anti- aging cream that contains Retinol. Retinol is a form of Vitamin A that has been shown to rejuvenate the effects of aging on the skin.

"B" is for blemish control. Blemishes, pimples, zits if you will, are not only for teenagers. They are something that can affect your skin for your entire life. So you need to always be diligent in your search for and treatment of blemishes and potential blemishes.

They can manifest themselves in a number of ways: whiteheads, blackheads, and minor inflammations. Each should be caught as early   as possible since they actually can be prevented   in most cases. If you can't stop them, you can conceal or cure them with over the counter medications and skin care products. What you use will vary depending on when you catch the blemish and what kind it is. Just be sure to use the proper medication rather than squeezing and popping your blemishes which can cause scarring and in some cases can even lead to more blemishes down the road.

"C" is for collagen. Collagen is contained in your skin and is what makes it elastic and smooth. As you age, the collagen molecules in the skin begin to break down .This break down creates wrinkles and lines on your face and body. The problem in the past has been that anti-aging creams could only use partial collagen molecules because they are large and difficult to get into the skin through lotion.

Recently, though, one major company developed and patented an infusion system for collagen. With it, creams can deliver whole collagen molecules into the skin. Once the collagen has been delivered, there is a noticeable difference. Your skin will have a healthy and rejuvenated glow. In addition, the wrinkles and lines that come with aging will begin to dissipate. Collagen is important, and it is the closest thing we currently have to a miracle aging cure.

If you are ready to put up a fight against the effects of aging, the process is going to start with your skin. Take the time to learn you're "ABC's" of skin care and you will start to look younger and your skin will begin to feel better. Remember, anti-aging cream, blemish patrol, and collagen is the key to your fight against aging skin.

CHAPTER 2- COMBINATION SKIN

Combination skin is when you have certain areas on your face that are dry and others that are oily.

Usually, the oily part of your face is in what is called the "t-zone" or the area of your forehead, nose and chin. When you have combination skin, you will probably notice that most days, you will experiences normal or dry skin. There are several ways you can take care of your combination skin. Here are six strategies for a healthy glow.

How can you be certain you have combination skin? If you have combination skin, your skin on your face might feel tight or dry after washing or taking a shower. Your face might also feel rough, look flaky or have an overall dull appearance. On the other hand, on other areas of your face, you will experience shiny skin that might feel or look greasy. This is most common in the "t-zone". Those areas are more prone to developing blackheads, pimples or other bumps.

There are ways to care for combination skin. After you have determined what kind of skin you have on your face, you can take steps to find the proper products and care for your skin. It may be that you have combination skin during certain seasons, such as summer. Your skin may be normal during other parts of the year. People, who spend a lot of time outdoors, might experience a dry skin all year round.

The first step you can take to treat and care for your combination skin is to cleanse. Look for products that are made specifically for combination skin and use it twice a day. This will help combat the oily skin on the "t-zone" and help keep other parts of the skin healthy. Make sure that you keep your face clean and free of residues at night. This is a good step to take towards caring for combination skin.

The second step to care for combination skin is to moisturize. When you have combination skin, some parts of your face might be oily, but other parts are dry and flaky. You cannot ignore the dry skin when treating the oily skin. The answer is to use moisturizer on the dry skin only. Products made for dry skin will help hydrate the dull and flaky skin. Try to keep the moisturizer off of the oily skin. That will only make it worse.

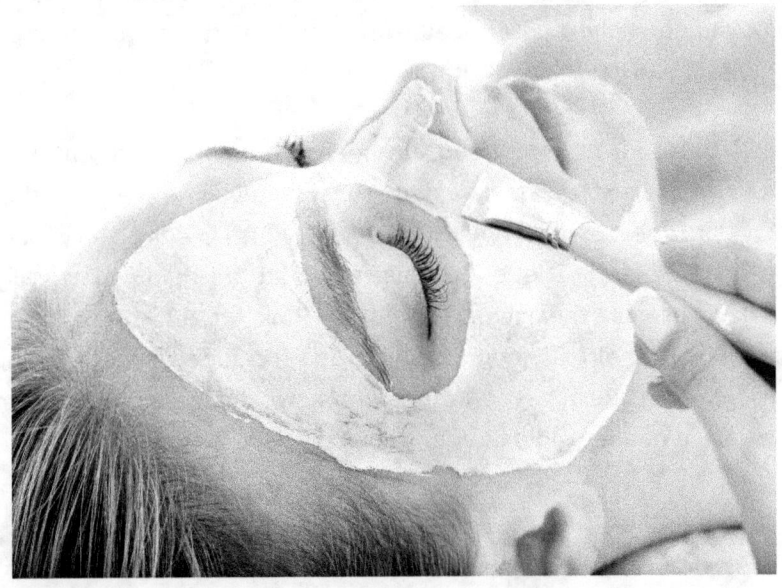

The third step is to balance your skin. There are many products that can help normalize your skin. Look for those that have alpha hydroxy acids, or retinol, which is a vitamin A product. Also, use a toner everyday to help keep the skin in balance. Steer clear of products that contain alcohol because that can irritate dry skin. Use toner at least once a week to combat combination skin.

How to Apply Make Up Like In the Movies

The fourth step is to control the skin by eating healthy and drinking plenty of water. When you practice a healthy diet, you can take a big step in controlling the quality of your skin. Fatty and greasy foods are not good for any type of complexion. Eat lots of fresh fruits and vegetables and try healthier oils. Drinking water will also help by hydrating your skin the natural way.

The fifth step is to use appropriate make up. Make up that contains oil-absorbing properties will help your appearance. Oil-free make up and make up that is labeled as non-comedogenic will help by minimizing the chances to pimples and blackheads. Another important part of skin care is to make sure make up is thoroughly removed each night before bed. Never go to bed with make up on because it can cause skin irritations.

The sixth step is to use a good sunscreen. Look for sunscreens with an SPF of at least 15. Using a daily sunscreen will help ensure that your skin does not become sunburned, which leads to dry skin. There are several varieties of sunscreen that are made specifically for daily use on the face. In addition, look for moisturizers and make ups that already contain sunscreen for added benefit. Using sunscreen every day, even in the winter, will help ensure   that you have a healthy glow to your skin.

CHAPTER 3- THE ART OF MAKEUP APPLICATION

Learning the correct techniques when applying make up can help you look your best. When you know what types of make up to use and how to properly apply them, you can make sure your appearance is always at its best. In addition to learning how to apply makeup, you should also understand what types of products are best for your skin type and what colors are most flattering to your complexion.

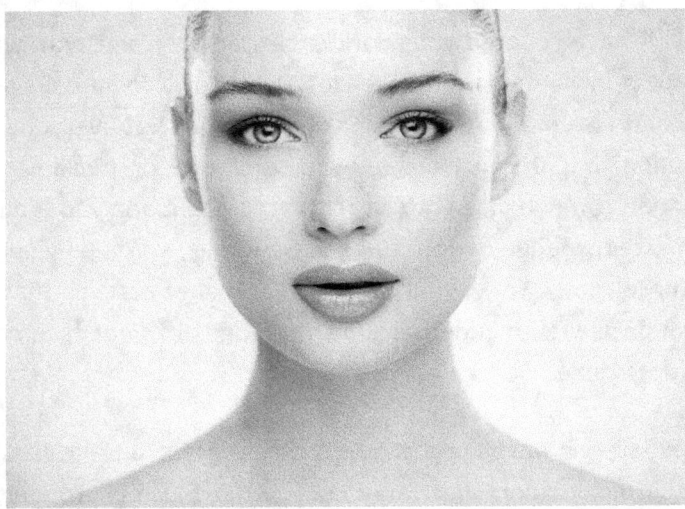

Applying makeup using the correct techniques does not have to be difficult or frustrating. There are two very common mistakes that women make when they apply makeup. They either use the wrong colors, or they apply too much make up. Using the wrong colors can make anyone look like they have just playing in their mother's make up bag.

How to Apply Make Up Like In the Movies

Generally, chose colors that compliment your skin tones. If you have light skin, do not go with dark colors. Also, do not try to apply too much make up. Apply just enough for a natural glow.

When you are ready to apply makeup, consider using a concealer. Concealer can help you hide under the eye circles, or flaws and blemishes on your skin. This can enhance the overall look of your face. Look for a concealer that closely matches your skin tone. If you get a color that is too light or too dark, it will show. When you apply the concealer, do not stretch the skin. Instead use a light patting motion. Concealer comes in stick creams, bottles and powders.

After you have covered your dark circles or blemishes you will be ready to apply foundation or base. This usually comes in a thin cream and also matches the color of your skin. Not everyone uses foundation, but if you have uneven skin tone or freckles, using foundation can enhance your appearance. When apply foundation, use a makeup wedge or your fingers. Generally, start applying from your nose and work your way out. Make certain that the foundation is well blended around the edges of your face so the line is not visible.

The next step in applying makeup is to use apply blush. Blush also comes in many colors and varieties. Powder blush is probably the most popular, followed by sticks or creams. Find a shade that compliments your skin tone. If you are applying the powder variety, use an angled make up brush and apply the powder on the apples of your checks. Brush the powder upwards towards your temples.

You can then blend in the powder using another brush. Make sure the blush is well blended around the temples making sure that the fine powder is not in the hairline.

After you have applied blush, you can apply the eye make up. Eye shadow can be a fun product to use if you want to experiment with different colors. Try shades until you find one that is flattering to you.

When applying eye shadows start at the corner of the eyelid and apply it going out. You can either use the applicator the make up comes with or use a small brush that will look like a flat paintbrush. You can then apply a lighter shade on the top of your eyelid and blend the two colors together. You can even experiment with using several shades together as long as you blend the colors together.

Now you can apply eyeliner and mascara. When you apply eye makeup, be careful to use clean applicators and never lick the eyeliner. Do not apply eyeliner on the inside of the eyelid. Eyeliner comes in various shades and in pencil form or a liquid form.

Pencil eyeliner is usually easier to apply than the liquid. Mascara also comes in several colors. If you have droopy eyelashes, consider using an eyelash curler for maximum effect. For those that suffer from watery eyes from allergies or who swim, look into using waterproof mascara.

When you are done, you can apply your lipstick. As a general rule, do not go to bright if you have pale skin. Make sure that you thoroughly remove all make up before going to bed each night. Also, throw away old make up when it is dry or cracked. Do not try to use old or expired make up, especially around the eye area.

CHAPTER 4- 50 MAKEUP TIPS

Choose Your Makeup Well

When you buy your makeup kit, make sure to choose something that is known for its quality. This way, you can be assured that you would be able to achieve the kind of effect that you are looking for. Aside from that, you can also ensure that you won't experience any kind of side effects on your skin with its use.

Consider Your Skin

In applying makeup, you need to make certain considerations to be on the safe side. For one, if your skin is allergic to certain types of makeup, then you should carefully select the makeup products you would apply on it. Aside from that, you should also consider your skin tone so that you can enhance your beauty with your makeup.

Consider Your Eyes

When you apply makeup, you should also consider your eyes. Keep in mind that there are certain makeup techniques used for women with deep set eyes as well as for those with regularly set eyes. By considering your eyes, you would be able to come up with a technique that can enhance it more.

Taking Care Of Your Makeup

There are certain makeup items, which should not be exposed to open air for a long period of time, since it can become brittle or are reduced in terms of quality. Therefore, you should make sure to close your makeup kit once you are done with it. Aside from that, you should store it in a place that is not too cold nor too hot.

Keeping Your Makeup Brushes

In most cases, when you are in a rush, you might end up living the brush you made use for your makeup by the mirror, or somewhere else. When you do this, you could experience having to look for it for hours the next time you want to use it. Thus, you should put it at the same place where you are usually keeping it, so that you can easily get it anytime you want.

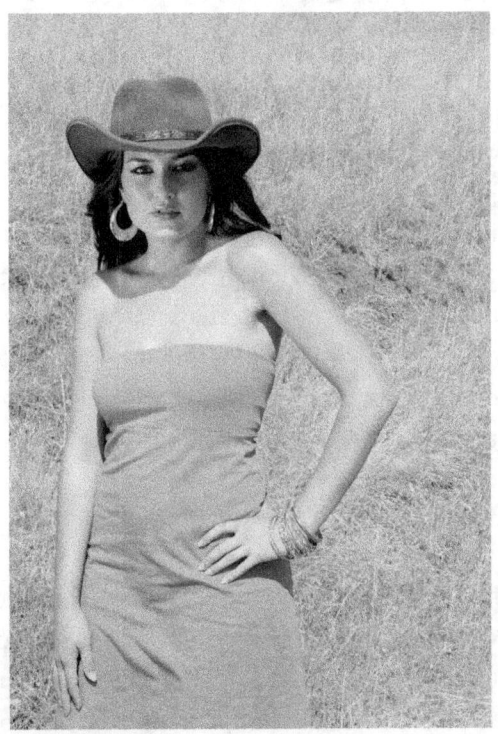

Saving Money with Makeup

If you want to make use of different shades of lipstick, manicures, pedicures, mascaras, and such, there is no need for you to buy them all. What you can do about it is to simply check out the makeup items of your friend. If you find something that you want to try, offer to swap it with yours or borrow it. You can also let her borrow some of yours to return the favor.

Don't Let Your Kids Play With Your Makeup

When you find that your daughters are playing with your makeup, you may find it amusing. However, you should not let them play with it, since you might end up with no makeup to use at all. Thus, you should keep your makeup items where your kids would not be able to reach it. Only let them use it, if you are around to monitor them.

Learning To Apply Makeup through the Internet

If you have just begun applying makeup, there are actually lots of things you can do for it. One of which is to search for the information that you need through the internet. All you have to do is to use your favorite search engine for it. Through the web, you can check out eBooks about the right way of applying makeup. Aside from that, videos are also available for you to access for free.

Hiring a Makeup Artist for Your Wedding

If you are in the process of hiring a makeup artist for your wedding, you need to see if she is really competent enough. One of the ways to do that is to check out her ideas about the makeup techniques she would use for you. It is very important that she comes up with a style that is fitted for your wedding theme, so that it would blend well with the whole get up.

Finding the Best Makeup Artists

To find the best makeup artists, one of the best ways to do it is through recommendations. You can actually call your friends, relatives, and even your colleagues to ask them about it. Once you

Jasinth H. Gooden

have gathered enough names and contact details, try calling some of them, and choose the one that you are most comfortable working with.

Have Fun

To become more effective in applying makeup on your face, you should see it as a fun activity. Don't put yourself down just because you are not able to perfect it on your first few attempts. Practice more, and be excited on the outcome, so that you will eventually improve your makeup skills.

Apply Makeup on Your Kids

To practice more in applying makeup, you should get your daughters involved in it. Try applying makeup on them, on certain occasions, so that you can also see your own progress. By doing that, you would be able to practice more, since you would be applying on someone else's face and not just yours.

Observe Makeup Artists Practice Their Skills

Whenever you visit the parlor, you should try to observe how various makeup artists apply their skills on their customers, in order to enhance their features. By doing this, you would be able to learn more about which shades go with what skin tones. Do this more frequently, and apply what you learn to yourself.

Establish Your Goals Well

In applying makeup, it is not just something that you have to do, simply because everyone is doing it. You need to have certain goals in mind, when you apply makeup. For instance, you should try to decide if you are applying makeup to enhance your eyes, nose, lips,

How to Apply Make Up Like In the Movies

or all of them. With certain goals on your mind, you can properly apply the right techniques in order to achieve them.

Visit Your Friends

Whenever you don't have anything to do on weekends, you should visit your friends, and practice applying makeup. Aside from providing you a chance to enhance your skills in it, you and your friends can also exchange ideas and tips about applying make up. Try it out this weekend, so that you can have some fun.

Use Your Imagination

If you are trying to design on the kind of style that you want to have in applying makeup, you should use your imagination for it. It is a good idea to not just stick on the basic techniques that you have learned through books and magazines. Try to explore new possibilities, since it may help you come up with newer techniques.

Read Magazines

To learn more about various makeup techniques, you can always read more magazines for it. This does not mean that you should limit yourself to reading the articles about applying makeup. You should also check out pictures of celebrities and see how their makeup experts enhanced their beautiful faces. By doing that, you can learn more about the various techniques that you can use on yourself.

Ask Questions

When you are in need of more information about applying makeup, you should ask more and more questions about it. There is no need to ask only one or two persons regarding this. You can ask your friends and relatives about it. Aside from that, whenever you visit a beauty salon and you are seated next to a makeup artist while waiting for your turn, then ask her questions, so that you can satisfy your hunger for information.

Check Out Blogs

Gone are the days when you need to step out of your place to acquire important information about applying makeup. You can simply do it by accessing the internet, and checking out blogs about it. Lots of blogs are launched with topics related to makeup.

Aside from offering informative articles, you can also post your questions on these blogs, which may be answered by the person behind it, or by other people who are visiting the site.

Start With Light Makeup

To be on the safer side, it is best that for your first few tries of applying makeup on yourself, you should do it lightly. With that, you won't have redo everything, when it comes out not the way you want it to be. Aside from that, it would also be easy to correct, since you won't be dealing with heavy makeup.

Applying Stage Makeup

If you are tasked to apply makeup on yourself for a stage play, you should keep in mind that it is entirely different to applying makeup for parties. For a stage play, your makeup should be something that can stand the hot lights, and be visible to people that are seated at the farthest row from the stage. However, you should also control it so that you won't look like a clown for people seated at the front row.

Makeup for Sensitive Skin

If you have sensitive skin, then it may take you some time to choose the makeup that won't get your skin irritated. Having allergic reactions from makeup is not something that you want to experience. To go around it though, you can always do a spot test prior to purchasing a product. This can be done by applying a small amount of the makeup on your skin. Wait 24 hours and see if you have any allergic reactions, before making up your mind.

Applying Makeup for Men

There is nothing wrong if a guy wants to apply makeup, especially if he only wants to cover certain imperfections. To do this, you can actually make use of the very basic makeup items. For example, to cover imperfections, you can use a concealer for that, and choose one that is a shade lighter than your skin.

Storing Your Makeup in the Bathroom

Storing your makeup inside the bathroom is not a good idea. This is because the bathroom is usually filled with a lot of moisture, which could be floating around midair. With this moisture would be bacteria and other germs, which can eventually get to your makeup, and affect its quality.

Using Sponges

If you like to use sponges in applying makeup, you should also take good care of it, aside from taking care of your other makeup items. The sponge should be washed clean every couple of times that you use it. If you want to make sure that you have a sponge that is top in quality every time you apply makeup though, you can always use a new one after using the sponge twice.

Washing Your Hands

It is important that you wash your hands thoroughly prior to using your makeup. This is to ensure that you won't get dirt on your makeup, as well as your face. If you find it such a hassle to go to the kitchen or bathroom to wash your hands though, you can always have a bottle of antibacterial lotion at the place where you are going to apply your makeup.

Store Makeup Testers

If you want to see if the color of the makeup would match your skin tone, or if you are allergic to it or not, you should avoid using the testers found in the stores. This is because they can harbor different types of diseases, and you might get affected of them just by trying them out. The best way to test a makeup is to visit a friend for it, or contact your makeup artist.

Makeup Hygiene

It is very important that you practice good makeup hygiene, since your makeup can make you visit your doctor soon. Some of the things that you need to take note of when it comes to this would be the proper storage of your makeup items, cleaning the brushes and sponges regularly, and many more. By practicing good makeup hygiene, you can prolong the life of your makeup items, and avoid going to the doctor due to it.

Infected Makeup

If you do get infected with a sort of disease, which you suspect came from your makeup; you should not be ashamed of it. You should still visit your doctor as soon as you can. If you experience allergic reactions, then take antihistamine, or call your doctor, so that you can take something that can provide you with immediate relief.

Using the Concealer

When you want to make use of a concealer to hide blemishes, pimples, or any other imperfections, there are things that you can do, in order to prolong its effects. One of which is to apply a light dusting on your face with loose powder. By doing that, you would be ensuring that the effects of the concealer would last for the whole night.

Using a Lip Balm

Lip balm can be used by both men and women, although some males hesitate using it, by thinking that it is unmanly. However, using a lip balm can actually help you in hydrating your lips. Therefore, when you use it in adequate amounts, you can prevent or take care of cracked lips.

Enhancing Your Lashes

If you are a guy and you want to look like a rocker or a hipster, then you should consider using an eyeliner. A black eyeliner pencil can help you a lot in achieving the looks that you want, by using it to line your upper and lower eyelashes. Choose a pencil that is really dark, so that you can really emphasize your lashes.

Using a Concealer for a Guy

Aside from making sure that the concealer you are using is of the right shade, it is also important to apply it at the right amount. If you don't want to look like you are indeed wearing makeup, then you should not apply too much of it. Aside from that, you should also make sure that you are applying it well so that you won't look like a pancake.

Choosing the Right Makeup

If you have experienced allergic reactions to some of your makeup items, one of the best ways to pinpoint the product that is causing it, is to check its labels. In most cases, one or some of your makeup items may contain allergenic ingredients. Once you are able to identify them, you should replace them with products that are safer to use, to avoid experiencing it again.

Applying Makeup on Your Kid, For Her School Play

When applying makeup on your daughter for her school play, start with a cream foundation, which has the same shade as her skin tone, or slightly darker. It should be paired up with blush on the cheeks. More importantly, use makeup items that are gentler on the skin, since your kid's skin is still very fragile.

The Loose Face Powder

Having a loose face powder on hand is important in applying makeup. One of its functions is to ensure that your makeup would stay in place longer. Aside from that, it can also ensure that the makeup won't melt in warmer temperatures. All you need to do is to apply it as a light dusting.

Shopping For Makeup for Your Kids

If you like applying makeup to your kids, then it is always best to go with milder items. To achieve that, when you shop around the malls, you should keep an eye out for makeup items that are hypo-allergenic, or at least fragrance free. By doing this, you can ensure that your kids' skin won't get irritated.

Organic Makeup

When you have sensitive skin, it is always best to wear makeup that won't irritate it, such as those that are made from organic ingredients. More and more products today are produced using organic materials, and these do not exclude makeup items. With an organic makeup, you can be assured that it is free from skin irritants like talc and dyes.

Lifespan of Your Foundation

The lifespan of your foundation can actually depend on the way that you use it. In most cases, if you use it with a pump, it can last for 8 months. However, if you are using it by dipping your fingers into the bottle, then you cannot expect it to go beyond the 6-month period.

Going Natural

Going for makeup kits that are made out of natural ingredients is actually a good idea, especially if you have sensitive skin. Aside from the fact that it can prevent skin irritation, it can also help in maintaining the health of your skin. This is because natural products do not contain synthetic ingredients, which are usually harmful to one's skin or body.

Pimples and Makeup

When you have pimples, using a concealer, especially something that has lighter shade than your skin can effectively hide it. To prevent pimples though, choose makeup items that are gentler on your skin. Such items usually do not contain substances that can clog up your pores and cause pimples.

Makeup for Healthier Skin

Keep in mind that your skin also needs minerals in order to remain as healthy as possible. With that, you should opt for mineral based makeup kits. By doing that, you are not just enhancing the beautiful features of your face, but, it can also improve the condition of your skin.

Applying Eye Makeup for the First Time

If it is going to be your first time to apply makeup on your eyes, then the best way to go about it is to use a pencil eyeliner. This is because pencil eyeliner is easier to work with, than the other kinds. Just make sure that you have a steady hand, so that you can do it perfectly.

Starting Out Fresh

When you are just starting to put makeup on your face, it is best to go with the basics first. A light foundation should help you a lot, but you should not apply it heavily at first. Aside from using a foundation, you can also utilize a concealer to hide the blemishes. Once you have gained more experience, then don't hesitate in exploring other makeup items.

Makeup for the Bride

Since it is going to be one of your most memorable days, you want everything to be perfect, including your makeup. Therefore, for your bridal makeup, you should not follow the trends, since they usually come and go, and you may not be sure if it would suit you best. Go for a more classic look, so that you would smile every time you check out your photos years after.

Makeup Colors for Your Wedding

To decide on the color of makeup you want to wear on your wedding, one of the things that you need to consider is your wedding theme. However, if you want to achieve that elegant look, stick with colors like pinks, browns, and plums, since they are soft to the eyes. Discuss this with your makeup artist, so that you would look your best on the big day.

Makeup Tips In Attending a Wedding

Knowing the wedding theme should be one of the first things that you should know before applying makeup on. This would ensure that you would be wearing the right dress and makeup color in attending the event. Aside from that, when you apply makeup, try to think about keeping your skin shine free, but glowing.

Wearing Makeup

Whatever kind of occasion your are attending to, you should make sure that you are wearing makeup that you are comfortable with. To achieve that, you should stick to makeup styles that are not too heavy. Aside from that, you should also choose makeup items that are non-allergenic.

Wearing Makeup at Work

When you wear makeup at work, you should stick to neutral colors, when it comes to your eyes. Earth tone eye shadows would look great with your office attire. For your eyeliner, you can choose one that has a gray or brown color to achieve that beautiful and professional look.

Enhancing the Looks of Your Lips

When it comes to your lips in reporting to work, you should stick to lighter shades of pink or red. This is because such colors are more professional than the other ones. Aside from that, you should avoid using lipsticks that are frost or have glittery effects. This can also apply to wearing lip gloss.

Chapter 5- 50 More Makeup Tips

Lifespan of Your Eye Shadow

When you purchase an eye shadow, you should choose one that is made by a reputable manufacturer. If you are able to do that, then you can expect it to last for a couple of years. However, you should also make sure that you store it properly, in which it is situated in a place that is not full of draft or moisture.

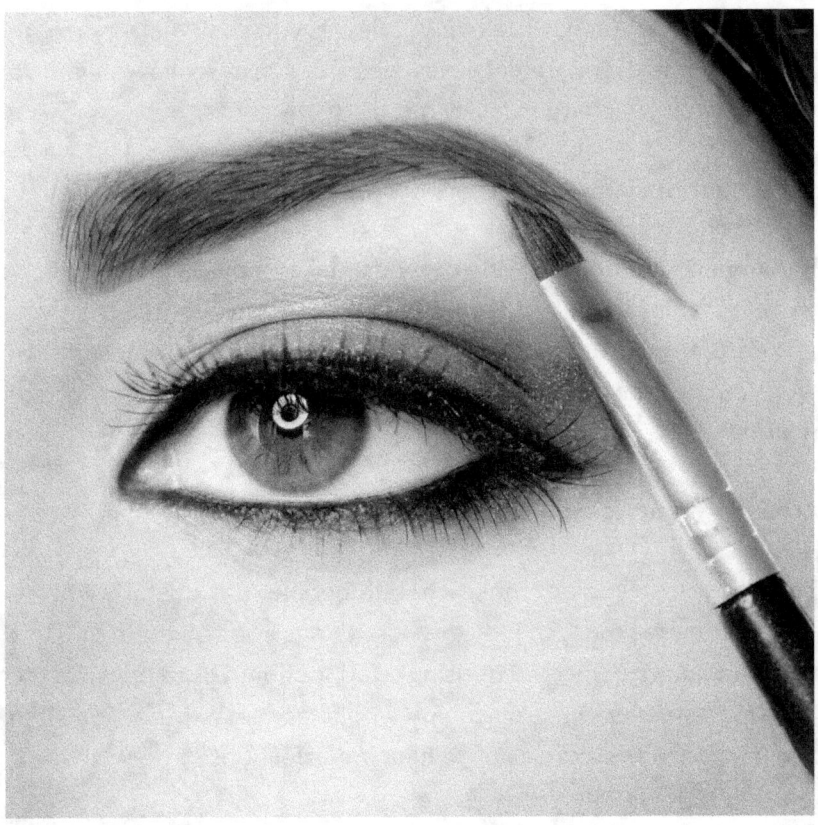

Lifespan of Your Mascara

Mascara is pretty much the same with a liquid liner, when it comes to its lifespan, which runs for only four months. Thus, it is best that you purchase a mascara wisely. If you can choose something that is a bit small, then you should stick to it, especially if you don't use mascara that much. Just make sure to close its container tightly, so that it won't get bad before consuming it all.

Lifespan of Lip Products

In most cases, most lip products, such as lipsticks and lip glosses can last for about 1 to 2 years. Storing it properly can ensure that it stays well until you use it all up. However, you should always try to check its smell. This is because, when it starts to have a rancid smell, then it is time to toss it out.

Open Your Makeup Purse Every Six Months

If you make it a point to open up our makeup purse once in every six months, in which you would take out all its contents, then you ensure that your makeup items are all fresh. This is because it can give you a chance to see which items are already done for, or are nearing their expiry dates.

Achieving That Natural Makeup Look

To achieve that radiant look, wherein people may mistake you for not wearing makeup, one of the best things you can do is to use a tinted moisturizer instead of using a foundation. This is because the tinted moisturizer will provide you with a less heavier look. Use it in conjunction with a concealer to hide imperfections.

A Good Way to Use Blush

If you use blush that is very close to your natural flush, then it can help you achieve the radiant look that you want. Aside from that, it can also make you look like you are not wearing any makeup at all. You can also use the blush to highlight your cheekbones to have that glowing look.

When to Wear Neutral Makeup

Neutral makeup simply means wearing light blushes, eye shadows that are in natural color, as well as neutral lip shades. This style of applying makeup is best worn for school or work. It is also the kind of makeup that you want to wear, if you are going to meet the parents of your boyfriend for the first time.

When to Wear Dramatic Makeup

Dramatic makeup means that you would be wearing red lips, smokey eyes, or simply dramatic combination of colors. This would be great for parties, as well as going out with your friends to discos or bars. Just make sure that you won't overdo it, so that people can still see your face.

Wearing Makeup Near Your Eyes

When you wear makeup just below your eyes, you need to be gentle with it. This is because the skin under your eye area is very sensitive. Thus, if you apply too much pressure on it, it can appear wrinkled or saggy. Just apply a little amount of makeup on it though if you want to, as long as you are conscious on how you are doing it.

Wearing Mascara and Eyeliner on Summer Months

If you want to wear mascara during summer, you should consider the fact that the heat can easily melt down your makeup. With that, it is best if you choose a waterproof mascara and eyeliner for your summertime look, so that you won't have to deal with smudges on the skin near your eyes.

The Best Way to Start In Applying Eye Makeup

The best way to apply eye makeup is to start with a clean skin. What you can do about it is to apply cold compress on your eyes for about 10 minutes. Doing this can actually reduce the puffiness of your eyes. After that, apply a light moisturizer so that the skin around your eyes, won't get dried up because of the makeup.

Styling Your Eyebrows

Some people tend to forget that one of the most important features of a person's face is her eyebrows. Therefore, you should assess it properly, so that you can apply the kind of style that would suit you best. One of the tools to style your brows is called the clipped-angle brush. Before using it though, determine the style that you want first, so that you can easily proceed.

The Eye Shadow Compact

Before making use of your eye shadow compact, make sure that you have already applied the foundation, or concealer to hide imperfections. If your eye shadow compact offers you three or four different shades, keep in mind that they are made that way, since you can actually use them together. Practice blending them though, before you attend parties so that you are assured that you are doing it right.

Applying Mascara

Using mascara can accentuate your eyelashes, especially if you are doing it the right way. To ensure that it is the case, when you apply mascara, you should slightly tilt your chin towards the top and lift your eyebrows. By following this position, you would be able to apply mascara without smearing.

Moisturizing Your Lips

Unless your lipstick is made to provide the needed moisture of your lips, you should make use of a lip balm prior to applying color on them. This practice can actually prevent chapped lips. Having chapped lips is not a pleasant experience, since it can become painful, especially if you are not able to take care of it immediately.

Applying Makeup While Having Pimples

If you have pimples and you want to apply makeup, it is actually fine. However, it is best if you go with gentler types of makeup items. This way, you won't be irritating your skin further. Aside from that, you should refrain from picking your pimples while using makeup, since it can worsen the situation.

Caring For Your Skin

If you are the type of person who usually wears makeup almost every day, then you should take care of your skin properly. One of the things you can do is to get a facial once a month. By doing this, your skin would be revitalized and purified. When that is achieved, it would become more radiant and won't get easily irritated with certain makeup items.

Your Daily Makeup

Wear a daily makeup that is simple and light, so that you won't put too much chemicals on your skin. Keep in mind that most makeup products are loaded with synthetic substances, which can harm your skin. Thus, it is best to stay on the safe side, and just use heavy makeup, when you are attending a party or going out with your friends.

Applying Foundation

When applying mineral or liquid foundation, it is best that you make use of a foundation brush. This way, you can ensure that you can balance the tones of your neck and your face. Choose a foundation brush that is made in good quality, and has flat and long bristles, so that you can apply foundation with ease.

Using The Right Face Brushes

It is important that you make use of the right types of brushes for every makeup item that is intended for your face. For example, a concealer brush is used for the concealer, so that you can properly hide pimples, and other imperfections. Aside from that, the blusher brush is used to color the cheeks. Use the proper brush, so that you can apply your face makeup properly.

Applying Makeup for the Eyes

The eyes are the windows of your soul; thus, you have to apply the right kind of makeup for it, so that it would help you express your feelings. You need to consider the color of your eyes, when it comes to choosing the shade of your makeup, so that you would be able to effectively enhance it.

Different Makeup Brushes

There are lots of different makeup brushes that you have to acquire in order to complete your makeup kit. These brushes are usually categorized depending on the part of the face they would be applied to. Some of them would be the face brushes, the lip brushes, the eye brushes, and some are called special brushes.

Jasinth H. Gooden
Choosing the Best Concealer

Aside from making sure that you are using the concealer that is lighter than your skin tone, there are other things that you need to consider for it. For instance, you should consider its brand, since there are certain brands that certainly stand out from the rest. Aside from the brands, you should also consider the type of concealer that you want.

The Advantages of Powder Concealer

There are lots of advantages in using a concealer that is in powdered form. For instance, it looks natural even at the end of the day. Aside from that, it would still provide you the effect that you want, even after you lay on a powder foundation. Moreover, it is also lightweight.

Using Liquid Concealer

If you want to hide some bad circles that are present under your eyes, then you want to make use of a liquid concealer. A liquid concealer is very easy to apply, since you can even use your fingers for it. Aside from that, it is very effective in hiding even the darker blemishes.

Choosing the Right Eye Shadow for Your Eyes

When choosing the color of your eye shadow, you should consider the color of your eyes. Thus, if you have blue eyes, then choosing the right shade of blue should help you enhance your beautiful eyes. To make sure that the shade perfectly matches your eye color, bring a friend with you when you shop for it.

Remove Your Makeup

How to Apply Make Up Like In the Movies

When you are about to go to bed, you should make it a practice to remove your makeup. This is to ensure that your skin won't get irritated with too much exposure to the substances that are present in your makeup. Aside from that, it can also ensure that your skin won't get dried out.

Wearing Eye Shadow to a Party

If you have just bought a new eye shadow to wear it for a party, you need to make sure that you are going to wear it with a dress that appropriately matches it. This is because the color of your dress can clash with the color of your eye shadow if you are not careful. Plan it well, so that you would look as stunning as you want to be.

Wearing Bright Makeup

If you are going to wear bright lips, bright cheeks, and bright eye shadow, then you may be overdoing it, and get your face covered with all our bright makeup. You need to achieve balance when wearing bright makeup. Thus, if you are wearing bright makeup for your eyes, then wear something neutral for your lips.

Achieving Beautiful Eye Makeup

To achieve a beautiful eye makeup effect, you need to have a concealer, eye shadow base, eye pencil, mascara, and eye shadow brushes. To achieve a more radiant effect, you need to use all these materials properly. Aside from that, you should also take note of the proper sequence in using them.

Explore

Once you have gotten more comfortable in applying makeup on your face, you should not be afraid in experimenting with different looks. By doing that, it actually provides you with more practice. Aside from that, it also gives you a chance to identify the best makeup style for your personality.

Finding the Most Affordable Makeup Products

If you want to find the most affordable makeup kits, what you can do is to explore the internet for them. Such kits are actually offered by various online stores in discounted prices. All you have to do is to find them through your search engine. To make sure that the makeup items are in good quality, don't forget to check out reviews about them.

Wearing Lip Liner If You Are a Guy

There is nothing wrong if you wear a lip liner if you are a guy, especially if you perform on stage. In fact, there are even real men who wear lipstick on a regular basis. If you want to try it out though, one of the things that you need to take note of, when buying the lip liner, is to choose something that is a bit darker than your normal lip color.

Preventing Eye Shadow from Creasing

Having a creasing eye shadow is not a pleasant experience. What you can do to prevent it is to make use of a reliable eye shadow primer. Choose one that is made by a reputable company, so that you are assured that your eye shadow won't fade. Aside from that though, a good primer can also make your eyes look more vibrant.

Enhancing Your Eyes with Concealer

A concealer is something that you can use to enhance your eyes aside from hiding your lower eye circles. Since the concealer can brighten up your eye area, your eyes would be emphasized. Just pair it up with mascara though, and curl up your eyelashes to provide you with a more youthful look.

Applying Dark Eyeliner Properly

Applying dark eyeliner can be tricky, since it can make your eyes look smaller if not done right. To make sure that you can emphasize the beauty of your eyes, the dark eyeliner should be applied on the lower lash line, instead of the inner rim of your eyes. Don't extend it to the inner corner, since it would make your eyes shrink.

Choosing Eye Shadow for Brown Eyes

Having brown eyes can make it easier for you to choose the color of your eye shadow, since that eye color can go with almost anything. However, if you want one that would suit your eye color best, then you should go with purple or green colored eye shadows.

Choosing the Right Type of Eye Shadow

When you are shopping for a new eye shadow, you need to be aware that they are available in different kinds. In general, eye shadows are available in cream, stick, powder, and mineral forms. Choosing between these kinds would depend on your preferences though, but it is also wise to know their differences.

The Shape of Your Eyebrow

Different haircuts go best with different women. This concept also applies to choosing the shape of your eyebrow. To determine the best eyebrow shape for you, one of the things that you can consider for it is the shape of your face. In general, faces can be oval, square, heart, or round shaped.

In Shaping Your Eyebrows

One of the things that you need to remember about shaping your eyebrows is that, they don't have to look like twins. They should look more like sisters, in which they should complement with each other. Aside from that, you should not over pluck since it can take some time to grow your eyebrows back.

Choosing Between Neutral and Dramatic Eye Shadows

Wearing eye shadow should be in accordance to the kind of event that you are attending. In general though, dramatic eye shadows should be worn during nighttime, especially on parties. On the other hand, neutral eye shadow should be worn for daytime such as at your office or at school.

What You Can Do With Thin Eyebrows

If you have thin eyebrows naturally or due to over plucking, you can make use of different types of eyebrow fillers for it. One example of it would be the eyebrow pencil, which you can use like you are drawing individual hairs, to compensate your lack of eyebrows. Don't apply too much pressure though, since it would appear unnatural.

Using Eyebrow Fillers

Whatever type of eyebrow filler you are going to use, it is very important that you match it with your hair color. However, if you have black hair, you should go for a dark brown color for your filler. This is because using black color could make your eyebrow look too harsh.

Having a Heart Shape Face

If your face is heart shaped, you should come up with rounded brows, since it would make your look more feminine and elegant. The rounded brows would emphasize your heart shape face. Whatever shape your face has though, it is best if you use an eyebrow gel in setting your brows.

How to Start Having a Winged Eyeliner

First and foremost, you should use a liquid liner to achieve the winged look. When it comes to applying it, it is good if you find a flat surface to rest your elbow on. This would help to steady your hand. Start at the inner side of your eye and get as close as you can to the lash line, while applying a line that is thin. This should help you in starting it right

Choosing the Right Kind of Eyeliner

One of the things you need to consider when choosing an eyeliner is its kind. The choices that you have would include the liquid eyeliner, pencil eyeliner, cream eyeliner, and mineral based eyeliner. It is best that you become more familiar with each of them, so that you can choose accordingly.

False Eyelashes

If you want to enhance the looks of your eyes by wearing false eyelashes, you should know certain things about them first. One of the things you need to take note of is the fact that most false eyelashes are too long for comfort. Thus, you may have to trim them down after purchasing them. Do it slowly though, so that they won't become too short.

Thickening Your Lashes with Mascara

Jasinth H. Gooden

There are different types of mascaras available today, and one of them can help you add more volume to sparse lashes. All you have to do is to choose mascara, which features a thickening formula to achieve what you want. Such products usually come with all the instructions that you need to follow.

Heated Eyelash Curlers

To curl your eyelashes, one of the things that you can make use of is the eyelash curler. However, if you want to speed things up, then you should opt for a heated eyelash curler. Such types of eyelash curler are usually battery operated, and have plates that would heat up when turned on. This tool would allow you to skip the step of heating up your curler in preparing it for the job.

ABOUT THE AUTHOR

Jasinth H. Gooden always dreamed of having her makeup done like the stars in Hollywood. She was so caught up with the art fo applying makeup that she transitioned form dressing up her dolls to applying makeup on her friends as a teenager to becoming a makeup artist as an adult.

She now works with those stars- helping to make them even more beautiful for their public appearances. She has published a book to help other makeup aficionados like herself to learn the proper techniques.

www.ingramcontent.com/pod-product-compliance
Lightning Source LLC
Chambersburg PA
CBHW061928280526
45787CB00004B/1518